ECZEMA HEALING DIET COOKBOOK

Unlocking Wellness: Delicious Recipes And Nutritional Guidance For Revitalizing Your Skin Naturally:

DR. SHAYLA LEWIS

Table of Contents

DISCLAIMER

Write a brief complete Disclaimer for my diet cook book telling them that the author is not in any association with any company, business or individual and also this book is written by the authors knowledge and understanding

The information provided in this diet cookbook is based on the author's personal knowledge and understanding. The author is not affiliated with, endorsed by, or associated with any company, business, or individual. The recipes and dietary advice contained within this book are intended for informational purposes only. Readers should consult with a healthcare professional or a registered dietitian before making any significant changes to their diet or lifestyle. The author assumes no responsibility for any adverse effects that may result from the use or misuse of the information contained in this book.

CHAPTER ONE

Understanding Eczema: An Overview

Eczema, commonly known as atopic dermatitis, is a persistent skin ailment marked by inflammation, itching, redness, and, in some cases, blistering. It frequently occurs as patches on the face, hands, feet, and other regions of the body. Understanding eczema requires a thorough understanding of its multidimensional nature, which includes genetic predispositions, immune system dysregulation, environmental triggers, and skin barrier malfunction. While eczema is not completely curable, proper treatment can greatly reduce symptoms and enhance quality of life. This necessitates a comprehensive approach that includes skincare, lifestyle alterations, and, most importantly, dietary changes.

Importance of Nutrition in Eczema Treatment
Nutrition is essential for managing eczema. The foods we eat can either aggravate inflammation or help the body heal. Certain dietary factors, such as food allergies or sensitivities, might cause eczema flare-ups in some individuals. In contrast, eating nutrient-dense meals high in vitamins, minerals, antioxidants, and essential fatty acids can help maintain skin health and minimize inflammation. Maintaining a healthy diet can also help to improve the immune system and promote general well-being, which is essential for managing eczema.

The advantages of a low-carb, antioxidant-rich, and anti-inflammatory diet are as follows:

Low-carb diets, such as the ketogenic diet, stress carbohydrate restriction while increasing the consumption of beneficial fats and proteins. This dietary strategy may benefit people with eczema because it helps to balance blood sugar levels and reduce inflammation, both of which are important in managing the illness. Antioxidant-rich diets emphasize foods high in antioxidants, such as fruits, vegetables, nuts, and seeds. Antioxidants help the body neutralize free radicals, which can contribute to eczema-related inflammation and oxidative stress. Similarly, anti-inflammatory diets focus on foods that help reduce inflammation, such as fatty fish, curcumin, ginger, and leafy greens. Individuals with eczema who adhere to these dietary rules may enjoy fewer flare-ups and better skin health.

How Diet Influences Nerve Pain and Symptoms

Diet can have a substantial impact on eczema-related nerve pain and symptoms.

Certain foods, such as processed sweets, refined carbs, and inflammatory fats, can worsen nerve pain and cause itching and discomfort. On the other hand, consuming foods high in omega-3 fatty acids, vitamins B12 and B6, and magnesium will assist in maintaining nerve function and reduce symptoms. Furthermore, maintaining stable blood sugar levels with a well-balanced diet will help minimize nerve pain spikes, which are frequently connected with blood glucose swings. Individuals suffering from eczema can enhance their general quality of life by paying attention to their food choices and their implications on nerve function.

Getting Started: Organizing Your Kitchen and Mindset

Setting up your kitchen and mentality for eczema healing entails both practical and psychological steps. Practically speaking, you should stock your kitchen with foods that promote skin health and inflammation reduction, such as fresh fruits and vegetables, lean meats, whole grains, and healthy fats. Purchasing high-quality cooking tools and utensils can also make meal preparation simpler and more fun. Equally crucial is developing a positive mindset and approach to eczema management.

This involves self-care, stress management strategies, and forming a support network of friends, family, and healthcare professionals who understand and empathize with your situation. You may empower yourself to take control of your eczema management by creating a supportive environment in your kitchen and in your head.

The Fundamentals of Eczema Healing

Eczema, also known as atopic dermatitis, is a chronic inflammatory skin illness distinguished by red, itchy, and inflamed patches of skin. It affects people of all ages, from infants to adults, and has a substantial impact on their quality of life. To avoid flare-ups, eczema patients must manage their symptoms, reduce inflammation, and identify triggers. This frequently necessitates a multimodal approach, including lifestyle adjustments, skincare routines, and dietary alterations.

What Are the Different Types of Eczema?

Eczema refers to a variety of skin disorders, with atopic dermatitis being the most frequent one. Contact dermatitis, dyshidrotic eczema, nummular eczema, and seborrheic dermatitis are among more kinds. Each variety has its distinct set of symptoms and triggers, but they all share the same feature of inflammation and itching. Understanding the type of eczema one has is critical for devising an effective treatment plan.

Identifying and avoiding triggers is critical for controlling eczema symptoms. Irritating soaps and detergents, allergens like pet dander and pollen, and specific foods like dairy, eggs, and gluten are all common triggers. Furthermore, environmental factors such as humidity and temperature fluctuations might aggravate symptoms. Individuals with eczema can lessen the frequency and severity of flare-ups by identifying and removing triggers.

The Role of Inflammation in Eczema

Eczema develops and progresses mostly because of increased inflammation. It is distinguished by an excessive immune response that causes redness, swelling, and itching of the skin. Chronic inflammation can weaken the skin barrier, leaving it more vulnerable to allergens and irritants. Managing inflammation is thus an important element of eczema treatment, which can be accomplished through a variety of methods, including topical creams, oral drugs, and lifestyle changes.

Understanding the gut-skin connection

Emerging evidence reveals a link between gut health and skin problems like eczema. The gut microbiome, which is made up of billions of bacteria that live in the digestive system, is essential for immune function and inflammatory regulation.

Gut microbiome disruptions, such as dysbiosis or leaky gut syndrome, have been linked to an increased risk of eczema and other inflammatory skin disorders. Individuals with eczema may benefit from boosting gut health through dietary changes and probiotic supplements.

CHAPTER TWO

The Value of a Holistic Approach to Healing

Healing eczema needs more than just treating the symptoms; it necessitates a multifaceted strategy that addresses the underlying causes of inflammation and immunological dysfunction. This involves eating a well-balanced diet rich in anti-inflammatory foods, using stress-management techniques, getting enough sleep, and maintaining a good skincare routine. Integrating complementary therapies such as acupuncture, herbal medicine, and mind-body practices can also help the body's natural healing processes.

Individuals who take a complete approach to eczema treatment can find long-term relief and enhance their overall health.

To summarize, managing eczema entails determining its causes, identifying triggers, and establishing a comprehensive treatment plan that addresses inflammation, gut health, and general wellness. Individuals who take proactive actions to assist their body's natural healing processes can effectively control their eczema symptoms and improve their quality of life.

Building Blocks of a Healing Diet

A healing diet for eczema focuses on providing the body with foods that enhance skin health, reduce inflammation, and promote internal healing. The components of such a diet include:

Fruits, vegetables, whole grains, nuts, seeds, and lean proteins are examples of entire, unprocessed foods to emphasize. These meals include critical elements such as vitamins, minerals, antioxidants, and fiber, which promote overall health and skin healing.

Choose nutrient-dense foods, which deliver a high number of nutrients per calorie. Leafy greens, berries, salmon, and sweet potatoes are some good examples. Nutrient-dense diets improve cellular function and aid the body's natural healing processes.

Balanced Macronutrients: Make sure your meals are balanced in terms of carbohydrates, protein, and healthy fats. Carbohydrates offer energy, protein aids in tissue repair and growth, while healthy fats reduce inflammation and promote skin integrity.

Variety: Include a wide variety of foods to ensure you get a diversified range of nutrients. Consuming a variety of fruits and vegetables guarantees that you receive a variety of vitamins, minerals, and phytonutrients that promote skin health and overall well-being.

Hydration: Keep yourself hydrated by drinking plenty of water all day. Proper hydration is vital for keeping the skin hydrated, aiding detoxification processes, and boosting general health.

Mindful Eating: Practice mindful eating by focusing on hunger and fullness indicators, as well as the sensory experience of eating. This can assist to prevent overeating and improve digestion and nutrient absorption.

Consistency is essential while following an eczema-healing diet. Make healthy eating a habit rather than a quick cure. Consistently nourishing your body with therapeutic foods can result in long-term skin health and overall well-being.

A Low-carb diet entails limiting carbs, particularly refined carbohydrates such as white bread, spaghetti, and sugary snacks while preferring whole, nutrient-dense foods. Low-carb eating may provide various possible benefits for those with eczema, including:

Reduced Inflammation: Refined carbs can cause inflammation in the body, which can worsen eczema symptoms. Individuals who reduce their intake of these inflammatory foods may experience fewer eczema flare-ups and general inflammation.

Low-carbohydrate meals can help stabilize blood sugar levels, which is beneficial for insulin management and minimizing the risk of insulin spikes and crashes. Stable blood sugar levels may lead to more consistent energy levels and less mood fluctuations, both of which can have an impact on eczema.

Weight Management: Low-carbohydrate eating may help overweight or obese people lose weight and manage their weight. Excess weight can cause inflammation and increase eczema symptoms, thus reaching a healthy weight may benefit skin health.

Increased Nutrient Intake: By focusing on full, nutrient-dense foods such as vegetables, fruits, lean proteins, and healthy fats, people who follow a low-carb diet can get more of the vitamins, minerals, and antioxidants they need for good skin and overall health.

Improved Gut Health: According to some research, low-carb eating may benefit gut health by limiting the consumption of potentially inflammatory foods and encouraging the growth of good gut flora. A healthy gut microbiota has been related to improved immune function, which may help alleviate eczema symptoms.

It's important to note that the effectiveness of a low-carb diet for eczema can vary from person to person, so consult with a healthcare physician or qualified dietitian to discover the best nutritional approach for your specific needs and preferences.

Adding Antioxidant-Rich Foods to Your Diet

Antioxidants are substances that assist the body in neutralizing damaging free radicals, which can damage cells and contribute to inflammation and other health problems, such as eczema. Adding antioxidant-rich foods to your diet can bring several benefits for skin health and overall well-being:

Protection from Oxidative Stress: Oxidative stress occurs when the body's free radicals and antioxidants are out of equilibrium, causing cellular damage. Antioxidant-rich foods assist to balance this imbalance by neutralizing free radicals and lowering oxidative stress, which may aid with eczema symptoms.

Anti-Inflammatory qualities: Many antioxidants have anti-inflammatory qualities, which can help reduce inflammation in the body and relieve symptoms of inflammatory disorders such as eczema. By including antioxidant-rich foods in your diet, you may notice fewer eczema flare-ups and general inflammation.

Skin Health Support: Antioxidants protect the skin from damage caused by environmental stresses such as UV radiation and pollution. They also aid in collagen formation, which is necessary for preserving skin suppleness and avoiding premature aging.

Immune System Support: Antioxidants like vitamins C and E are believed to improve the immune system. A robust immune system is critical for general health and may help to lessen the frequency and severity of eczema flare-ups.

Fruits (such as berries, citrus fruits, and grapes), vegetables (such as leafy greens, bell peppers, and carrots), nuts and seeds, legumes, and some spices (such as turmeric and cinnamon) are all rich in antioxidants. Including a variety of these items in your diet will help guarantee that you obtain a wide range of antioxidants to promote skin health and overall well-being.

Incorporating antioxidant-rich foods into your diet is a simple yet effective strategy to boost eczema healing and overall wellness. To increase your antioxidant consumption, incorporate a range of colorful fruits and vegetables, nuts, seeds, and spices into your meals and snacks.

CHAPTER THREE

Anti-inflammatory foods and their benefits

Inflammation is a normal immunological reaction that aids the body in fighting infection and healing injuries. Chronic inflammation, on the other hand, can lead to the onset and worsening of a variety of health disorders, including eczema. Adding anti-inflammatory foods to your diet can help reduce inflammation and relieve eczema symptoms:

Omega-3 Fatty Acids: Omega-3 fatty acids are found in fatty fish such as salmon, mackerel, and sardines, as well as flaxseeds, chia seeds, and walnuts. They have significant anti-inflammatory qualities. They help reduce inflammation in the body and promote skin health, making them beneficial to people who have eczema.

Turmeric's main ingredient, curcumin, is known for its significant anti-inflammatory properties. Including turmeric in your diet or drinking turmeric tea can help reduce inflammation and alleviate symptoms of inflammatory disorders such as eczema.

Leafy Greens: Dark leafy greens such as spinach, kale, and Swiss chard are high in antioxidants and anti-inflammatory chemicals, which assist the body combat inflammation. Consuming these greens can improve general health and may help decrease eczema flare-ups.

Berries, including blueberries, strawberries, and raspberries, are high in antioxidants and flavonoids, which have anti-inflammatory qualities. Including berries in your meals or as a snack can help reduce inflammation and improve skin health.

Ginger includes gingerol, a chemical that has powerful anti-inflammatory and antioxidant properties. Including fresh ginger in your meals or drinking ginger tea will help reduce inflammation and relieve symptoms of inflammatory disorders such as eczema.

Green tea contains polyphenols, which have powerful antioxidant and anti-inflammatory properties. Drinking green tea on a regular basis can help reduce inflammation in the body and promote general health, including skin health.

Incorporating these anti-inflammatory items into your diet will help reduce inflammation, improve eczema symptoms, and boost overall health. To maximize the benefits for skin health and immunological function, incorporate a range of these foods into your meals and snacks.

The Strength of Hydration and Healthy Fats

Hydration and good fats are essential for skin health and overall well-being, particularly for people with eczema. Understanding their significance and adding them to your diet can help reduce eczema symptoms and promote healing.

Hydration: Proper hydration is necessary for maintaining skin moisture and suppleness, which is especially critical for eczema patients who may have dry, itchy skin. Drinking plenty of water throughout the day keeps the skin hydrated from the inside out and promotes its natural barrier function.

Healthy Fats: Omega-3 fatty acids, found in fatty fish, flaxseeds, and walnuts, are essential for skin health and inflammation regulation. These fats help preserve skin moisture, reduce inflammation, and improve overall skin integrity, making them beneficial to eczema sufferers.

Avocado contains monounsaturated fats, vitamins E and C, and antioxidants, all of which benefit skin health and moisture. Avocado in your meals or snacks can help keep your skin hydrated and lessen the likelihood of eczema flare-ups.

Coconut oil includes medium-chain fatty acids that are hydrating and anti-inflammatory, making it good for people who have eczema. Applying coconut oil directly or incorporating it into your recipes will help relieve dry, irritated skin and reduce inflammation.

Olive oil contains monounsaturated fats and antioxidants, which help reduce inflammation and promote skin health. Using olive oil as a salad dressing or in cooking will help keep your skin moisturized while also promoting internal healing.

Nuts and seeds, like almonds, walnuts, and chia seeds, are high in healthy fats, vitamins, and minerals that promote skin health. Including a variety of nuts and seeds in your diet can help to keep your skin hydrated and minimize irritation.

Hydration and healthy fats are vital for improving skin health and relieving eczema symptoms. Drink plenty of water throughout the day and incorporate healthy fats into your meals and snacks to keep your skin moisturized and nourished from the inside.

Creating Balanced Meal Plans for Eczema Relief

To create balanced meals for eczema relief, include a variety of nutrient-dense foods that support skin health, reduce inflammation, and improve overall well-being. Here are some recommendations for preparing balanced meals that can help decrease eczema symptoms.

Include Lean Proteins: Lean proteins like chicken, turkey, fish, tofu, and lentils include important amino acids that help with tissue repair and growth. Protein in your meals helps you feel full and promotes skin healing.

Vegetables are high in vitamins, minerals, antioxidants, and fiber, all of which help to maintain skin health and overall well-being. To increase nutritional intake and improve satiety, fill half of your plate with non-starchy veggies such as leafy greens, broccoli, carrots, and bell peppers.

Incorporate Healthy carbs: Whole, unprocessed carbs such as quinoa, brown rice, sweet potatoes, and whole grains provide long-lasting energy and critical nutrients. Avoid refined carbs such as white bread, pasta, and sugary snacks, as they can cause inflammation and worsen eczema symptoms.

Include Healthy Fats: To support skin health and reduce inflammation, incorporate healthy fats into your meals, such as avocados, nuts, seeds, and olive oil. A drizzle of olive oil on salads or avocado slices in sandwiches might assist in keeping your skin hydrated and nourished.

Stay Hydrated: Drink plenty of water throughout the day to stay hydrated and moisturize your skin. Hydrating solutions for eczema-related dry skin include herbal teas, coconut water, and infused water with fresh fruits or herbs.

Mindful Eating: Practice mindful eating by focusing on hunger and fullness indicators, as well as the sensory experience of eating. Eating slowly, chewing properly, and savoring each bite will help you avoid overeating while also improving digestion and nutritional absorption.

Limit Trigger Foods: Identify and avoid foods that cause eczema flare-ups or worsen existing symptoms. Dairy, gluten, eggs, soy, and processed meals containing artificial additives and preservatives are all common triggers. Keeping a food journal can help you recognize patterns and make informed decisions about which foods to include or exclude.

You may improve skin health, reduce inflammation, and relieve eczema symptoms by eating balanced meals that include lean proteins, plenty of veggies, nutritious carbohydrates, and vital fats. Experiment with different recipes and ingredients to see what works best for you, and reap the advantages of a healthy diet for an eczema cure.

Diet has a significant impact on whether eczema symptoms worsen or improve. A nutrient-dense diet can assist promote the body's natural healing process while also reducing eczema inflammation. This section of the Eczema Healing Diet Cookbook has a variety of nourishing meals intended to promote skin health and overall well-being.

These dishes incorporate nutrients renowned for their anti-inflammatory effects, such as omega-3 fatty acids found in fatty fish like salmon and mackerel, as well as antioxidants prevalent in fruits and vegetables. Including these foods in your diet will help soothe inflamed skin and minimize the frequency and severity of eczema flare-ups.

From substantial soups loaded with bright veggies to savory salads rich with vitamins and minerals, each meal has been carefully crafted to provide a balance of critical elements to support skin health. Whether you're looking for comforting classics or inventive dishes, these healthy recipes provide great options for individuals seeking eczema relief through dietary adjustments.

CHAPTER FOUR

Breakfast ideas to start your day

Starting your day with a nutritious breakfast sets the stage for good health and well-being. Breakfast can be an opportunity for those with eczema to ingest items with skin-nourishing effects

This section of the Eczema Healing Diet Cookbook contains a range of breakfast recipes meant to get your day started with great flavors and healing ingredients.

From creamy porridge with fresh berries to vitamin and mineral-packed smoothie bowls,

41

each recipe is designed to deliver long-lasting energy while also boosting skin health. Nuts, seeds, and leafy greens are high in vital fatty acids and antioxidants, which can help reduce inflammation and speed up skin healing.

Whether you favor sweet or savory breakfast alternatives, these dishes provide innovative ways to integrate eczema-friendly products into your morning routine. Fueling your body with nutritional foods in the morning will help your skin's natural healing process and improve your general well-being.

Healthy Lunch Ideas for Long-Lasting Energy:

A nutritious lunch is critical for maintaining energy levels throughout the day, especially for people with eczema. This section of the Eczema Healing Diet Cookbook contains a range of nourishing lunch meals meant to create a nutritional balance to promote skin health and overall wellness.

Each recipe, from brilliant salads filled with leafy greens and colorful veggies to hearty grain bowls packed with protein and fiber, provides a fulfilling and nourishing dinner. Lean proteins, whole grains, and leafy greens are high in vitamins, minerals, and antioxidants, which can aid in reducing inflammation and promote skin healing.

Whether you're meal-prepping for the week or having a relaxing lunch at home, these recipes offer tasty ways to fuel your body with eczema-friendly ingredients. Incorporating nutrient-dense ingredients into your midday meals will help your skin's natural healing process and keep you feeling energized all day.

Snacking can be a good way to get more nutrients during the day, especially if you have eczema. This section of the Eczema Healing Diet Cookbook contains a selection of nutrient-dense snack foods that will give you an energy boost while also supporting your skin's health.

From handmade energy bars filled with nuts and seeds to crunchy veggie sticks combined with creamy hummus, each recipe provides a delightful and gratifying snack. Nuts, seeds, and fruits are high in vital fatty acids, vitamins, and minerals, which can help reduce inflammation and speed up skin healing.

Whether you're seeking something sweet or spicy, these snack recipes offer quick and nutritious ways to satiate hunger between meals. By selecting nutrient-dense snacks prepared with eczema-friendly foods, you can help your skin's natural healing process and maintain overall wellness.

A nutritious dinner is critical for replenishing nutrients and promoting overall health, especially for people with eczema. This section of the Eczema Healing Diet Cookbook contains a selection of tasty dinner recipes that will nourish your body while also improving your skin's health.

From hearty stews with vegetables and lean proteins to savory stir-fries with herbs and spices, each recipe provides a filling and nutritious meal option. Fish, poultry, whole grains, and leafy greens are high in important nutrients, which can help reduce inflammation and promote skin healing.

Whether you're cooking for yourself or eating with loved ones, these dinner dishes offer imaginative and savory ways to integrate eczema-friendly items into your evening meals. Prioritizing nutrient-dense foods at dinner will help your skin's natural healing process while also providing delicious meals that nourish the body from the inside out.

Satisfying your sweet taste does not have to mean jeopardizing your health, especially for those with eczema. This portion of the Eczema Healing Diet Cookbook contains a variety of desserts and snacks that will satisfy your desires while also boosting your skin's health and overall well-being.

From luscious avocado chocolate mousse to refreshing fruit sorbets, every recipe provides a delightful and guilt-free way to satisfy your sweet tooth. Avocado, coconut milk, and fresh fruits add natural sweetness while also being high in vitamins, minerals, and antioxidants, which can help reduce inflammation and promote skin healing.

Whether you're celebrating a special occasion or simply craving something sweet, these dessert dishes provide innovative and nutritious alternatives to classic treats. You can enjoy delectable sweets without jeopardizing your health or increasing eczema symptoms by selecting desserts produced with eczema-friendly ingredients.

CHAPTER FIVE

Meal planning was made simple

Meal planning is an important part of treating eczema with diet. It entails planning your meals ahead of time to ensure you're eating foods that support healing while minimizing stressors. The Eczema Healing Diet Cookbook is a thorough guide to making this process easier, with practical ideas and delicious meals designed to relieve eczema symptoms.

First, meal planning entails discovering and adding eczema-friendly foods into well-balanced meals. These foods often include anti-inflammatory elements such as fruits, vegetables, lean meats, and healthy fats. The cookbook explains which foods are excellent for eczema recovery and includes a variety of recipes for incorporating them into everyday meals.

Furthermore, the cookbook highlights the significance of a varied diet. You can guarantee that you obtain all of the required vitamins and minerals for skin health by choosing meals that include a variety of nutrients and flavors. The cookbook's recipes are intended to be varied and savory, making it simpler to maintain your eczema-healing diet over time.

Furthermore, meal planning takes into account cooking time, convenience, and dietary constraints. The cookbook provides advice for effective meal preparation and proposes batch cooking specific items to save time on hectic days. By planning meals ahead of time and keeping items on hand, you can avoid the temptation to choose less healthful options when time is of the essence.

Overall, the Eczema Healing Diet Cookbook makes meal planning easier by providing clear instructions on how to select eczema-friendly foods, prepare balanced meals, and maximize kitchen convenience. You can use it to create a long-term food planning habit that will aid you on your path to better skin.

Understanding Portion Control for Eczema Management.

Portion control is important in eczema management since certain foods might worsen symptoms or cause flare-ups. The Eczema Healing Diet Cookbook teaches readers the importance of portion control and offers ways for properly managing food consumption to promote skin health.

Understanding proper serving sizes for various food groups is an important element of portion control. The cookbook provides portion size advice for various cuisines to help readers prevent overconsumption of potentially harmful substances. Individuals who follow this advice can improve their calorie control and maintain a balanced diet that promotes eczema healing.

Furthermore, portion management is more than just managing the amount of food ingested; it also includes mindful eating practices. The cookbook advises readers to pay attention to hunger cues, eat carefully, and relish every bite. Individuals who practice mindful eating can create a healthy relationship with food and lower their risk of overeating.

The cookbook also offers practical portion management recommendations, such as using smaller plates, measuring quantities with kitchen equipment, and avoiding distractions when eating. These tactics can assist individuals in becoming more aware of their food intake and making deliberate choices to support their eczema treatment goals.

Furthermore, portion control is vital for keeping a healthy weight, which is necessary for eczema treatment. Individuals can lower the risk of obesity-related comorbidities that can aggravate eczema by limiting their calorie intake. The cookbook emphasizes the importance of portion control in reaching and maintaining a healthy weight as part of a holistic eczema management strategy.

In conclusion, understanding portion control is critical for efficient eczema management through nutrition. The Eczema Healing Diet Cookbook offers readers helpful ideas and practical tips for navigating portion sizes, developing mindful eating habits, and supporting their road to healthy skin.

Weekly Meal Prep Tips and Tricks

Weekly meal preparation is a game changer for people with eczema because it ensures they have access to nutritional meals throughout the week while reducing the temptation to eat less healthy foods. The Eczema Healing Diet Cookbook contains useful tips and tactics for quick and successful food preparation, allowing readers to take charge of their diet and achieve their skin health goals.

One of the primary advantages of weekly meal planning is that it saves time and effort on busy weekdays. Individuals who devote a few hours on the weekend to prepare meals and snacks for the week ahead can streamline their cooking process and reduce the stress of picking what to eat each day. The cookbook includes step-by-step instructions for planning and carrying out a successful meal prep session, from recipe selection to ingredient and container organization.

The cookbook also includes suggestions for maximizing freshness and flavor when preparing meals ahead of time. This includes employing correct storage procedures, such as airtight containers and labeling things with expiration dates, to ensure that food is safe to eat throughout the week. Individuals who follow these guidelines can retain the quality and nutritional value of their cooked meals.

Furthermore, the cookbook advises batch cooking as a time-saving method for meal preparation. Individuals can quickly build a variety of meals throughout the week by preparing large batches of staple foods such as cereals, meats, and sauces rather than starting from scratch each time. This technique not only saves time but also encourages dietary variety and flexibility.

Furthermore, the cookbook emphasizes the necessity of meal planning using eczema-friendly ingredients for better skin health. Individuals can improve their eczema management diet by selecting meals that include anti-inflammatory foods and avoiding typical irritants. The cookbook includes a plethora of recipes specifically created for meal planning, ensuring that readers have access to delicious and wholesome meals all week.

In conclusion, weekly meal preparation is a strong tool for eczema patients, and the Eczema Healing Diet Cookbook provides readers with the knowledge and resources they need to implement this practice effectively. Individuals who follow its suggestions and tactics can save time, reduce stress, and improve their skin health by eating nutritious and simple foods.

Adapting Recipes to Suit Your Dietary Needs

Individuals with eczema must adapt recipes to meet their specific dietary demands because certain components can cause flare-ups or worsen symptoms. The Eczema Healing Diet Cookbook emphasizes the significance of customization and includes instructions for changing dishes to meet different dietary choices and limits.

One of the most important components of adjusting recipes is replacing products that may be harmful to eczema with suitable substitutes. Individuals with dairy sensitivity, for example, can replace cow's milk in recipes with plant-based alternatives such as almond or coconut milk. Similarly, gluten-free flours can be used as a substitute for wheat flour to suit persons who are gluten-sensitive.

Furthermore, the cookbook recommends avoiding or eliminating items that are recognized as eczema triggers, such as processed sugars, artificial chemicals, and common allergies. Individuals can make these changes to produce dishes that meet their nutritional demands while remaining delicious and enjoyable.

The guidebook also includes suggestions for modifying seasonings and flavors to suit particular tastes. This could include limiting salt consumption, utilizing alternative herbs and spices for seasoning, or experimenting with different cooking techniques to enhance the natural flavors of ingredients. Individuals can enjoy a wide variety of meals that cater to their taste preferences while also supporting their eczema treatment goals by personalizing recipes in this manner.

Furthermore, the cookbook promotes culinary creativity and flexibility, allowing readers to modify recipes based on product availability and personal tastes.

Individuals can customize recipes to meet their specific nutritional needs and culinary preferences, whether it's substituting veggies in a stir-fry or including alternative proteins in a salad.

In conclusion, adjusting dishes is an important skill for eczema patients, and the

Eczema Healing Diet Cookbook offers practical advice on personalizing meals to meet specific nutritional needs. Individuals can enjoy delicious and nutritious meals that complement their skin health goals by making deliberate item substitutions, changing seasonings, and being creative in the kitchen.

Budget-Friendly Strategies for Healthy Eating Maintaining a healthy diet while treating eczema does not have to be expensive. The Eczema Healing Diet Cookbook provides cost-effective techniques and tips to help people make nutritious food choices without going overboard.

The cookbook recommends meal planning and batch cooking as a cost-saving method. Individuals can prevent food waste and the need for costly last-minute purchases by planning meals in advance and cooking large batches of essential foods. Batch cooking also allows for bulk purchasing of ingredients, which is frequently less expensive than purchasing smaller quantities.

Furthermore, the cookbook highlights the necessity of wise purchasing and using inexpensive foods. This includes choosing seasonal fruit, purchasing generic brands, and buying products in bulk or on sale. Individuals who are clever about grocery shopping can stretch their food budget while still eating a range of nutritional meals.

The cookbook also includes advice for repurposing leftovers and using materials wisely to reduce waste. For example, leftover veggies can be repurposed in soups or stir-fries, and cooked grains can be used as a base for salads or grain bowls. Individuals can save money and lessen their environmental impact by making the most of their ingredients.

Furthermore, the cookbook advises on how to prioritize spending on high-quality, nutrient-dense meals that help with eczema control. While some specialty items may be more expensive, investing in nutrients like fresh fruits, vegetables, and lean proteins can result in better skin health and general well-being.

In conclusion, the Eczema Healing Diet Cookbook offers realistic suggestions for eating healthily on a budget, allowing individuals to prioritize their skin health without going overboard. Readers can enjoy nutritious and budget-friendly meals that help them manage their eczema by adding meal planning, smart purchasing practices, and ingredient efficiency into their routine.

CHAPTER SIX

How to Overcome Common Meal Planning Challenges

Meal planning can be quite beneficial for people living with eczema, but it is not without obstacles. The Eczema Healing Diet Cookbook acknowledges these challenges and provides suggestions to assist readers overcome typical barriers to good meal planning.

Finding time to plan and prepare meals is a typical difficulty, especially for people who have busy schedules. The cookbook recommends making meal planning and grocery shopping a weekly priority. Individuals who prioritize meal preparation can guarantee that they have nutritious meals available throughout the week, even during busy times.

Furthermore, the cookbook offers suggestions for streamlining and improving the meal planning process. This includes meal planning templates or applications, establishing uniform grocery lists, and batch-cooking specific dishes to save time during the week. Individuals who implement these organizing tactics can simplify meal planning and lessen their likelihood of feeling overwhelmed.

Furthermore, the cookbook covers the issue of dietary constraints and preferences within a household. It provides tips on how to accommodate varied dietary demands while still eating together as a family. This could entail establishing common ground with flexible recipes that can be tailored to different preferences, or preparing distinct components to fit certain dietary constraints.

The cookbook also acknowledges the urge to deviate from the meal plan when confronted with unforeseen circumstances or cravings. It urges readers to be flexible and forgiving, acknowledging that occasional deviations from the plan are common and should not jeopardize long-term success. Individuals who follow a balanced approach to meal planning and allow for flexibility can overcome frequent problems and maintain consistency in their eczema management journey.

To summarize, meal planning presents certain hurdles, but the Eczema Healing Diet Cookbook offers practical ideas to assist readers overcome these obstacles. Individuals can build a long-term meal planning practice that supports their skin health goals by dealing with time constraints, dietary restrictions, and the desire to break from the plan.

Dining out and managing social situations can be especially difficult when you have eczema. However, with some practical advice and methods, you can enjoy these activities without jeopardizing your dietary demands or causing flare-ups.

To begin, make a plan ahead of time. Before going out, look into restaurants in your region that provide eczema-friendly options or are prepared to meet dietary requirements. Many places now cater to a variety of dietary demands, including gluten-free, dairy-free, and even eczema-specific requests.

When assessing meals, prioritize basic, whole-food choices. Look for recipes containing lean meats, including grilled chicken or fish, as well as plenty of veggies. Avoid foods that are highly processed, fried, or contain recognized eczema triggers such as dairy, gluten, or too much sugar.

Tips for Navigating Restaurant Menus with Eczema

Navigating restaurant menus with eczema in mind necessitates a sharp eye for products and cooking processes. Begin by examining the menu for probable allergens, such as dairy, gluten, nuts, and soy. Many restaurants now include allergen information on their menus or provide separate allergy menus upon request.

When in doubt, ask your server about ingredient substitutes or changes. Most places are happy to accommodate dietary restrictions in order to provide a pleasant eating experience for all guests. For example, you can ask for olive oil instead of dairy-based sauces or gluten-free bread or pasta.

Dining out with eczema requires effective communication. Communicate your dietary requirements to your server or restaurant personnel, and don't be hesitant to ask questions about how foods are made. It is critical to advocate for yourself and ensure that your meals are free of any potential triggers.

When discussing your dietary limitations, be polite but firm, and give clear directions to help the kitchen staff better understand your demands. To avoid cross-contamination, you can request that your dish be cooked without specific components or prepared separately.

Strategies for Attending Social Gatherings Without Stress

Attending social gatherings with eczema can be unpleasant, especially if food is an important part of the event. However, with proper planning and methods in place, you may confidently manage these scenarios.

Before attending a social function, contact the host to discuss your dietary requirements. Offer to bring a dish that you know is safe to eat, so you have at least one option. Consider having a small, balanced meal before the event to satisfy hunger and reduce the temptation to eat trigger foods.

During the event, concentrate on mingling rather than just the food. Engage in talks, activities, and socializing with others. If food is served, take the time to thoroughly consider your options and select those that meet your nutritional needs.

Making Informed Choices at Parties and Events

When attending parties and events, making smart food selections is critical for eczema treatment. Begin by inspecting the buffet or appetizer table to discover dishes that are safe to eat. Search for fresh fruits and vegetables, lean proteins, and whole grains.

Be cautious of portion amounts and avoid overeating trigger foods. Choose smaller amounts of dishes that may include possible triggers, or try sampling a little piece to see how your body reacts. Also, drink plenty of water throughout the event to stay hydrated and promote good skin.

If you have any questions regarding the ingredients of a particular meal, please ask the host. It's best to err on the side of caution and avoid foods that may aggravate your eczema symptoms.

CHAPTER SEVEN

Maintaining balance while eating out is critical for treating eczema and improving Aoverall health. While it is vital to be aware of trigger foods and make informed decisions, it is also ok to indulge sometimes and in moderation.

Include a variety of nutrient-dense foods in your diet, such as fruits and vegetables, whole grains, and lean proteins. These foods contain important vitamins, minerals, and antioxidants that promote good skin and immunological function.

When eating snacks or dining out, practice portion control and pay attention to your body's hunger and fullness cues. Avoid restricted or too rigorous eating habits, as they can cause feelings of deprivation and contribute to stress and anxiety.

Remember that managing eczema involves not only what you eat, but also how you care for your skin and overall health. Incorporate stress-relieving activities into your routine, prioritize sufficient sleep, and stick to your skincare regimen to aid healing and prevent flare-ups.

Supplements and Extra Support

When it comes to managing eczema through food, supplements can help to improve skin health and reduce inflammation. However, before introducing any new supplements to your routine, you should proceed with caution and contact a healthcare expert.

Essential fatty acids, including omega-3 and omega-6 fatty acids, are an important issue. These are essential for maintaining proper skin function and decreasing inflammation.

Fish oil supplements, which are high in omega-3 fatty acids, have been researched for their possible benefits in eczema treatment. Similarly, some studies have suggested that evening primrose oil, which includes gamma-linolenic acid (GLA), an omega-6 fatty acid, can help reduce eczema symptoms.

Probiotics are another important dietary supplement to consider. Probiotics are helpful bacteria that improve gut health, influencing immune function and inflammation. According to some studies, certain probiotic strains may help alleviate eczema symptoms, particularly in children.

Vitamin D is also required for skin health and immunological function. Some studies have revealed a link between vitamin D insufficiency and eczema severity, although further study is needed to substantiate this hypothesis. Nonetheless, maintaining enough vitamin D levels through supplementation or sunlight exposure may be advantageous to general skin health.

Other supplements worth investigating are zinc, vitamin E, and quercetin, all of which have antioxidant characteristics and may help reduce eczema-related inflammation.

However, it is critical to note that supplements are not a substitute for a nutritious diet and lifestyle. They should be used in conjunction with a holistic strategy for eczema therapy, which may include dietary changes, skin care, stress management, and maybe medication, depending on the severity of the symptoms.

Essential Supplements for Eczema Healing
Certain nutrients stand out as eczema healing supplements due to their ability to support skin health and reduce inflammation. Omega- fatty acids, found in fish oil

supplements, are among the most well-known and thoroughly studied. These essential fatty acids have anti-inflammatory effects and may help treat eczema symptoms by lowering inflammation in the body.

Evening primrose oil is another popular supplement among eczema patients. It contains gamma-linolenic acid (GLA), an omega-6 fatty acid that may lower inflammation and improve skin barrier function.

Probiotics are becoming more widely known for their ability to promote gut health and modulate the immune system. According to some studies, certain probiotic strains may help alleviate eczema symptoms, particularly in children.

Vitamin D is required for proper skin health and immunological function. While more research is needed to completely understand the association between vitamin D and eczema, some people may benefit from supplementing or getting enough sunlight.

Zinc is another vitamin that influences skin health and wound healing. Some studies suggest that zinc supplementation may help lessen eczema symptoms, but additional study is needed to substantiate these findings.

Vitamin E is an antioxidant that may help protect the skin and prevent inflammation. While evidence on vitamin E for eczema is limited, it may be effective as part of a comprehensive skin health regimen.

Quercetin is a flavonoid present in several foods, including apples, onions, and green tea, as well as supplements. It has antioxidant and anti-inflammatory effects and may help alleviate eczema symptoms by regulating the immune system.

Before beginning a new supplement regimen, consult with a healthcare expert to identify the best method for your specific needs. They can assist you in assessing your nutrient status, identifying potential drug interactions, and developing a supplement plan that compliments your overall eczema care strategy.

Consider Herbs and Natural Remedies

In addition to dietary adjustments and supplements, many eczema patients look into herbal cures and natural treatments to help manage their symptoms. While research on herbal therapies for eczema is limited, several herbs and natural substances have shown promise in terms of lowering inflammation, calming irritated skin, and improving overall skin health.

Chamomile is a popular eczema treatment plant. Chamomile has anti-inflammatory and anti-itch qualities, making it an ideal treatment for irritated skin. It can be applied topically in the form of creams or ointments, or taken internally as a tea.

Calendula is another herb that is often used to treat eczema. It has anti-inflammatory and wound-healing effects and may help lessen the redness and itching that accompany eczema flare-ups.

Aloe vera is well-known for its soothing and hydrating characteristics, making it a favorite choice among eczema patients. Aloe vera gel helps moisturize dry, irritated skin while also reducing inflammation.

Licorice root extract has been investigated for its possible use in eczema treatment. It contains anti-inflammatory qualities and, when applied topically, may help relieve itching and redness.

Oatmeal baths are a traditional treatment for eczema and other skin problems. Oatmeal includes chemicals known as avenanthramides, which have anti-inflammatory qualities and can help soothe irritable skin when used in bathwater.

Coconut oil is another natural treatment that some people find beneficial for eczema. When applied to the skin, it has hydrating characteristics and may aid in the reduction of inflammation.

While these herbal cures and natural treatments may provide relief for some people, they should be used with caution and in consultation with a healthcare practitioner before incorporating them into your eczema management strategy. They should be used as part of a comprehensive eczema care plan that includes dietary adjustments, stress management, and, if necessary, medical treatment.

Consulting with Healthcare Professionals for Personalized Advice

When it comes to managing eczema with diet and lifestyle modifications, consultation with healthcare specialists is critical for individualized advice and direction.

While there is a multitude of information regarding eczema healing diets on the internet and in books, it is critical to seek advice from trained doctors who can customize a plan to your specific needs and circumstances.

A dermatologist or allergist can help you identify and prevent eczema triggers, such as particular foods, environmental allergens, or skincare products. They may also recommend drugs or topical therapies to help manage flare-ups and prevent infections.

A trained dietitian or nutritionist can help you create a diet plan that promotes skin health and lowers inflammation. They can help you identify foods that can cause eczema flare-ups and propose nutrient-dense diets that promote healing and overall well-being.

Other healthcare specialists may also be involved in your eczema treatment strategy.

A mental health counselor or therapist, for example, can assist you in developing stress-relief techniques and coping strategies to deal with the emotional effects of living with a chronic skin condition.

It is critical to talk freely and honestly with your healthcare provider about your eczema symptoms, treatment objectives, and any concerns or questions you may have. Working together, you can create a complete eczema management strategy that addresses all aspects of your health and well-being.

Implementing Stress-Relief Techniques into Your Routine

Stress has been shown to be a significant trigger for eczema flare-ups in many people. As a result, adding stress-relieving activities into your daily routine can be an important part of effectively controlling eczema. There are several stress-relief treatments available, and determining which one works best for you may need some experimentation.

Mindfulness meditation is a popular stress-relieving method. Mindfulness is the practice of paying attention to the present moment without passing judgment, which can help reduce stress and promote relaxation. Many people find that simply a few minutes of mindfulness meditation per day can improve their overall sense of well-being.

Deep breathing exercises are another helpful stress reduction approach. Deep breathing activates the body's relaxation response, which can offset the physiological effects of stress. Deep breathing can be practiced by inhaling deeply through your nose, holding for a few seconds, and then slowly expelled through your mouth.

Progressive muscle relaxation is another strategy for stress reduction and relaxation. Tensing and then gently releasing each muscle group in your body, beginning with your toes and progressing to your head. This can assist to decrease stress and produce a state of serenity.

Yoga, tai chi, spending time in nature, listening to music, writing, and spending time with loved ones are all stress-relieving techniques that may help manage eczema. Experiment with different approaches to determine which one works best for you, and then include them in your daily routine to help manage stress and lessen the likelihood of eczema flare-ups.

It's also critical to address any underlying stressors in your life, such as work, relationships, or financial issues. This may entail changing your lifestyle or obtaining help from a mental health expert.

Incorporating stress-relief practices into your routine and addressing sources of stress in your life can help lessen the frequency and severity of eczema flare-ups while also improving your general quality of life.

Tracking progress and adjusting your approach as needed.

Tracking your success is an important part of managing eczema with diet and lifestyle modifications. By keeping track of your symptoms, nutrition, skincare routine, and other factors, you can spot patterns and triggers that may be causing your eczema and make necessary changes.

A symptom diary is one method for keeping track of your progress. This entails documenting your eczema symptoms, such as itching, redness, and flare-ups, as well as any triggers, such as certain meals, environmental allergies, or stressors. Keep track of your symptoms and any dietary or lifestyle changes with a notepad, smartphone app, or internet tool.

Tracking your dietary intake can also help you identify potential triggers for eczema symptoms. Keep a food journal and make a note of any foods that appear to increase your symptoms. You may also wish to consult a trained dietitian or nutritionist to help you identify and eliminate trigger items from your diet.

In addition to recording your symptoms and nutrition, it's critical to consider other things that may influence your eczema, such as skincare products, environmental allergies, and stress levels. Keep track of any changes you make to your skincare routine or environment, as well as their effects on your symptoms.

As you track your progress, be willing to make changes to your strategy as needed. If you notice that particular foods or environmental variables appear to aggravate your eczema symptoms, attempt to avoid or limit your exposure to them. If you're not getting the outcomes you desire, consult a healthcare professional to help you identify potential triggers and create a more effective treatment strategy.

You can control your eczema and enhance your general quality of life by tracking your progress and making necessary modifications. Remember that managing eczema is an ongoing process, and it may take some time to find the technique that works best for you. Be patient with yourself and remain committed to your health and well-being.

When it comes to managing eczema, food modifications are frequently the initial step, but lifestyle changes are equally important in achieving long-term health. Lifestyle modifications affect many parts of everyday life, including physical activity, sleep patterns, stress management, and the creation of a supportive atmosphere

CHAPTER NINE

The importance of regular exercise for eczema management

Regular exercise not only benefits overall health but also helps to manage eczema symptoms. Exercise increases blood circulation, which helps to deliver necessary nutrients to the skin and remove toxins, supporting skin health. Furthermore, physical activity reduces stress, which can cause eczema flare-ups. However, it is critical to select low-impact exercises and avoid activities that may result in excessive sweating or skin irritation. Incorporating activities such as yoga, swimming, or brisk walking into your daily routine can bring both physical and emotional advantages while not worsening eczema symptoms.

Quality sleep is essential for skin restoration and overall well-being, particularly for eczema sufferers. During sleep, the body, especially the skin, heals and regenerates. A lack of sleep can weaken the immune system and promote inflammation, resulting in more frequent and severe eczema flare-ups. To increase your sleep quality, stick to a consistent sleep schedule, develop a soothing nighttime routine, and make sure your sleeping environment is comfortable. Meditation, deep breathing exercises, and the use of relaxing essential oils can all help to relax and improve sleep quality.

Stress and Its Effect on Eczema Symptoms

Stress is a significant cause of eczema flare-ups and can exacerbate current symptoms. Learning good stress management skills is critical for treating eczema and promoting general health. Incorporating mindfulness techniques like meditation, yoga, or tai chi can help reduce stress and increase relaxation. Additionally, indulging in hobbies or activities you enjoy can give a much-needed distraction from tensions while also contributing to mental well-being. It is also critical to prioritize self-care and seek assistance from friends, family, or a therapist if stress gets excessive.

Creating a Healing Environment

Creating a supportive environment is critical for treating eczema and fostering healing. This encompasses both the physical and emotional aspects of the environment. Make sure your living space is free of any irritants or allergens that could cause eczema flare-ups, such as harsh detergents, pet dander, and dust mites. To reduce your exposure to potential triggers, purchase hypoallergenic mattresses, clothing, and skincare items. In addition, surround yourself with a supporting network of friends and family who understand your situation and can offer encouragement and aid as needed.

Embracing Self-Care Practices for Overall Wellness

Individuals with eczema must prioritize self-care because controlling the condition can be physically and emotionally demanding. Practicing self-care can assist to reduce stress, increase mood, and promote general well-being. This involves prioritizing activities that bring you joy and relaxation, such as spending time outside, performing hobbies, or taking a warm bath. It's also critical to care for your skin by following a moderate skincare routine, hydrating regularly, and avoiding harsh chemicals or scents that can irritate it. Remember to pay attention to your body's demands and prioritize self-care as an important aspect of your eczema management strategy.

In summary, lifestyle modifications are essential for controlling eczema and maintaining long-term wellness. Individuals can effectively manage their symptoms and enhance their overall quality of life by combining regular exercise, putting sleep first, controlling stress, creating a supportive atmosphere, and embracing self-care techniques.

Answering Common Concerns and FAQs

Eczema is a chronic inflammatory skin disorder that can have a substantial influence on one's quality of life. When it comes to diet-based eczema management, several typical issues and queries occur. Let's tackle a few of these:

Understanding Triggers: Many people who have eczema are curious about which foods or environmental variables cause flare-ups. While triggers differ from person to person, frequent food sensitivities include dairy, gluten, eggs, nuts, and some fruits. Harsh soaps, synthetic materials, and pollen can all act as environmental triggers.

nutrition and Eczema: There is emerging evidence that nutrition is important in treating eczema symptoms. Certain foods can promote inflammation in the body, causing flare-ups, whilst others may have anti-inflammatory characteristics that can help relieve symptoms.

Elimination Diets: Elimination diets entail removing potential trigger foods from your diet for a period of time before gradually returning them to see which ones exacerbate your symptoms. This procedure can be difficult, but it is often effective in identifying triggers and developing a specific eczema-friendly diet plan.

Nutritional Deficiencies: People frequently worry about whether removing specific foods from their diet would result in nutritional deficiencies. It is critical to ensure that your eczema healing diet is balanced and contains all of the important nutrients. Consulting with a healthcare physician or nutritionist might assist you in creating a nutritious food plan.

Lifestyle Factors: In addition to food, stress, lack of sleep, and environmental allergies can all have an impact on eczema symptoms. Addressing these variables holistically is essential for effective eczema care.

Long-Term Strategies: Many people worry if making dietary adjustments alone will bring long-term relief from eczema. While nutrition can play an important role, it is frequently only one part of a complex approach to eczema management. Long-term success requires consistency, patience, and continual monitoring.

When starting an eczema healing diet, it's necessary to contact healthcare professionals such as dermatologists, allergists, and dietitians. They can offer individualized advice based on your specific needs and medical history.

By addressing these common concerns and queries, people can feel more equipped to manage the intricacies of managing eczema with dietary treatments.

Dealing with Flare-ups: Quick Relief Tips

Flare-ups are an unpleasant part of life with eczema, producing discomfort and, in some cases, suffering. While a comprehensive eczema healing diet can help prevent flare-ups, it is critical to have methods in place to deal with them when they do develop. Here are some strategies for immediate relief.

Moisturize: Keeping the skin moist is essential for treating eczema flare-ups. To lock in moisture, apply moderate, fragrance-free moisturizers or emollients on a regular basis, particularly after bathing.

Cool compresses: Applying cool, moist compresses to the affected region can help relieve irritation and inflammation. Avoid using hot water because it can irritate the skin more.

Topical therapies, such as corticosteroids or calcineurin inhibitors, are available over the counter or on prescription and can provide relief from itching and irritation during flare-ups. Follow your healthcare provider's advice regarding their use.

Avoid Scratching: Although it may be tempting to scratch affected areas, doing so can aggravate irritation and cause additional skin damage. Keep your nails short, and try wearing cotton gloves at night to reduce itching while sleeping.

Identify Triggers: Consider what foods, skincare products, or environmental factors may have prompted the flare-up. Avoiding these triggers may help to prevent future flare-ups.

Stress Management: Stress is a known trigger for eczema flare-ups, so stress-reduction practices like deep breathing, meditation, or yoga may help ease symptoms.

Stay moisturized: Drinking enough water keeps your skin moisturized from the inside out, which can help reduce inflammation and promote healing.

Seek Medical Advice: If home remedies do not provide significant relief or if the flare-up is severe, contact your doctor. They can suggest additional medication alternatives or make changes to your eczema management plan.

By implementing these methods into your eczema treatment routine, you will be able to properly address flare-ups and reduce their influence on your everyday life.

CHAPTER TEN

Natural Relief for Itching and Discomfort

Eczema's defining symptoms are itchiness and irritation, which can cause severe misery and interfere with daily activities. While numerous drugs are available to treat these symptoms, many people prefer to try natural alternatives. Here are some natural ways to reduce the irritation and pain caused by eczema:

Oatmeal baths can relieve itching and inflammation. Colloidal oatmeal, which is widely available in pharmacies, can be mixed with lukewarm bathwater to relieve sensitive skin.

Coconut oil is known for its hydrating and anti-inflammatory characteristics, making it a popular natural eczema cure. To nourish and soothe itchy skin, use virgin coconut oil straight to the affected areas.

Aloe Vera: Aloe vera gel, generated from the aloe vera plant's leaves, offers cooling and soothing characteristics that can help alleviate eczema. To relieve irritation and inflammation, apply pure aloe vera gel to the affected regions.

Cold compresses or ice packs can provide instant relief for itchy skin by numbing the region and lowering inflammation. To avoid making direct touch with the skin, wrap the ice pack in a thin towel.

Calendula, often known as marigold, contains anti-inflammatory and antibacterial qualities that can relieve eczema-prone skin. Look for creams or ointments containing calendula extract and apply to the affected areas as needed.

Probiotics: Some evidence suggests that probiotics, which promote a healthy balance of gut flora, may help alleviate eczema symptoms such as itching. It may be useful to eat probiotic-rich foods like yogurt, kefir, and sauerkraut, as well as take probiotic supplements.

Mind-Body Techniques: Because stress can increase eczema symptoms, practicing relaxation techniques like deep breathing, meditation, or progressive muscle relaxation can help manage itching and pain.

Avoid Triggers: Identify and avoid things that aggravate your eczema symptoms, including particular meals, harsh skincare products, and environmental allergies.

While natural therapies can be successful for mild to moderate eczema symptoms, it is critical to check with a healthcare practitioner before attempting any new treatment method, especially if your symptoms are severe or chronic.

Coping with the Emotional Challenges of Living with Eczema

Living with eczema may be taxing not just on the physical but also on the mind, as the condition can impair self-esteem, social interactions, and quality of life. Coping with the emotional issues of eczema necessitates strength and support. Here are some ways to deal with the emotional side of living with eczema:

Education and Awareness: Understanding eczema and its triggers can help decrease the worry and anxiety that comes with the condition. Learn about eczema management tactics, treatment alternatives, and ways to reduce flare-ups.

Communicate freely with friends, family, and healthcare providers about how eczema affects you physically and emotionally. Expressing your feelings and concerns might help others understand your needs and offer assistance.

Prioritize self-care activities that promote relaxation and well-being, such as meditation, yoga, spending time in nature, or indulging in enjoyable hobbies. Taking care of your mental and emotional health is critical for dealing with the symptoms of eczema.

Set Realistic Goals: Set specific goals for controlling your eczema, focusing on little changes you can take every day to enhance your symptoms and quality of life. Celebrate your accomplishments, no matter how modest, and be patient with yourself when you face setbacks.

Professional Help: If eczema-related stress, anxiety, or despair become overpowering, consult a therapist or counselor. Therapy can provide a safe area to explore and manage the emotional impact of having eczema.

Positive Self-Talk: Question negative attitudes and beliefs about yourself and your eczema. Exercise self-compassion and remind yourself that eczema does not define your worth or identity.

Focus on What You Can Manage: While you may not be able to entirely manage your eczema, you can control certain parts of your life, such as maintaining a healthy lifestyle, controlling stress, and pursuing effective treatment choices.

Coping with the emotional difficulties of eczema necessitates a combination of self-care methods, social support, and expert assistance. Prioritizing your mental and emotional well-being allows you to better manage the impact of eczema on your life and thrive in the face of obstacles.

While traditional medical treatments are frequently beneficial in managing eczema, some people may seek alternative or complementary therapies to support their treatment regimen. These alternate ways may bring additional benefits or relief to people who prefer natural therapies. Here are some alternative therapies and treatments for eczema:

Acupuncture, a traditional Chinese medicine method in which small needles are inserted into particular places on the body, may help alleviate eczema symptoms such as itching and irritation. Some research indicates that acupuncture can alter the immune system and improve skin barrier function.

Herbal Medicine: Teas, tinctures, and topical creams containing herbs such as chamomile, calendula, and licorice root have been used for millennia to treat a variety of skin diseases, including eczema. However, there is limited data to support their usefulness for eczema, therefore they should be used with caution.

Homeopathy is a holistic treatment technique founded on the premise of "like cures like," in which very diluted medicines are used to promote the body's self-healing capabilities. Individual symptoms and constitution may dictate which homeopathic medicines are advised for eczema.

Traditional Chinese medication (TCM) views eczema as an imbalance in the body's interior environment, with the goal of restoring equilibrium through procedures including acupuncture, herbal medication, nutritional therapy, and qigong.

Gut health is important for immune function and inflammation, thus ingesting probiotics (beneficial bacteria) and prebiotics (fiber that feeds gut bacteria) may help alleviate eczema symptoms by fostering a healthy gut microbiota.

Essential oils, such as lavender, tea tree, and chamomile, offer anti-inflammatory, antibacterial, and calming characteristics that may help with eczema-prone skin. Dilute essential oils in a carrier oil and apply topically to problematic regions, or use aromatherapy diffusers to relax.

Mind-Body Practices: Mind-body practices including meditation, yoga, tai chi, and biofeedback can help reduce stress, which is a significant cause of eczema flare-ups. These activities, which promote relaxation and emotional well-being, may supplement conventional eczema therapies.

Dietary Supplements: Fish oil (omega-3 fatty acids), vitamin D, and evening primrose oil have all been researched for their possible advantages in treating eczema symptoms. More study is needed to determine their efficacy and safety.

Before attempting any alternative or complementary therapy for eczema, you should contact a healthcare expert, especially if you are currently using prescription medications or have underlying health concerns. They can provide advice on safe and effective treatment alternatives that are suited to your specific needs.

Finding Community and Support for Your Eczema Journey

Living with eczema can feel isolating at times, but finding community and support can make a big difference in your path to recovery and acceptance. Whether you're looking for practical help, emotional support, or simply a sense of belonging, connecting with others who understand what you're going through may be empowering. Here are some methods to discover community and support throughout your eczema journey:

Attending eczema-related conferences, workshops, or seminars can help you learn more about the condition, treatment options, and self-care practices. These gatherings also offer the opportunity to network with healthcare experts and other eczema warriors.

Advocacy Organizations: Join eczema advocacy organizations or patient advocacy groups that increase awareness, promote research, and advocate for better treatments and support services for eczema patients.

Therapy and Counseling: To address the emotional burden of having eczema, consider pursuing individual or group therapy. A qualified therapist can offer you support, coping methods, and a safe space to discuss your thoughts and concerns.

Family and Friends: Surround yourself with supporting family members and friends who will listen, encourage you, and guide you through the ups and downs of life with eczema. Open communication and understanding might help to improve your support network.

Be an Advocate: Share your eczema experience with others in an open and honest manner in order to raise awareness and minimize stigma around the condition. By speaking out and advocating for yourself and others with eczema, you may contribute to a more supportive and inclusive community.

Finding community and support along your eczema journey is critical for emotional well-being, empowerment, and resilience. Connecting with others who understand and empathize with your experiences, whether online or in person, can bring comfort, validation, and encouragement as you face the challenges of living with eczema.

Monitoring Progress and Celebrating Success
Tracking progress and celebrating achievement are essential parts of any healing journey, especially when dealing with illnesses like eczema. These components are especially important in an eczema healing diet cookbook because they provide actual evidence of the efficacy of dietary adjustments and their effects on symptom management.

CHAPTER ELEVEN

Before beginning any of the dietary modifications indicated in the eczema healing diet cookbook, it is critical to set baseline measurements so that progress may be reliably tracked. These metrics could include the severity and frequency of eczema flare-ups, the extent of irritation and inflammation, and general skin health. Baseline measurements serve as a benchmark against which progress can be tracked over time.

Individuals may utilize proven eczema severity scoring systems, such as the Eczema Area and Severity Index (EASI) or the Scoring Atopic Dermatitis (SCORAD) index, to measure the severity of their symptoms at the start of their dietary intervention. In addition, they may photograph damaged regions in order to physically track changes in the appearance of their skin.

The food and symptom notebook is an important tool in the recovery path through dietary therapy. This journal is a complete record of daily dietary consumption and any eczema symptoms that occur. Individuals who painstakingly track their meals, snacks, beverages, and symptom occurrences can find patterns and probable triggers that exacerbate their eczema.

Individuals are instructed in the eczema healing diet cookbook context to note not only what they consume, but also the timing of meals, portion quantities, and any accompanying symptoms such as itching, redness, or swelling. This method enables the identification of specific foods or food groups that may be associated with flare-ups, allowing for targeted dietary changes to help with symptom management.

Recognizing Non-Scale Victories on the Way:

While dietary therapies are often designed to improve eczema symptoms, it is also vital to acknowledge and appreciate non-scale triumphs along the road. Non-scale triumphs include any beneficial results that go beyond decreases in eczema severity or symptom frequency. These victories may include increased energy, better sleep quality, higher mood, or a greater sense of overall well-being.

Non-scale successes in the context of an eczema-healing diet cookbook may take the form of increased confidence in managing one's disease, the capacity to efficiently recognize and navigate food triggers, or a renewed appreciation for healthy, eczema-friendly meals. Celebrating these accomplishments promotes the value of overall well-being and provides an incentive to continue prioritizing dietary treatments for eczema management.

Celebration of Milestones and Achievements

As people advance through their eczema healing journey, it's critical to celebrate milestones and accomplishments to recognize their hard work and dedication. Milestones may include meeting particular symptom improvement targets, successfully applying nutritional suggestions from the cookbook, or maintaining good lifestyle changes over time.

Milestones can be celebrated in a variety of ways, from modest acknowledgments of accomplishment to more major awards or self-care gestures. This could include rewarding oneself with a favorite activity, indulging in a spa day, or sharing accomplishments with loved ones for additional encouragement and support. Individuals who commemorate milestones reconfirm their dedication to their health and eczema control goals.

Staying Motivated in the Face of Obstacles and Setbacks

Plateaus and setbacks are unavoidable parts of every healing path, including those aimed at treating eczema with dietary changes. During these difficult times, it is critical to remain focused and resilient in the pursuit of long-term health. The eczema healing diet cookbook focuses on efficient ways to negotiate plateaus and failures, ensuring that people stick to their nutritional goals.

Key strategies for staying motivated during plateaus and setbacks may include revisiting the initial reasons for starting the healing journey, seeking support from healthcare professionals, peers, or online communities, and adjusting dietary strategies based on newfound insights or changing needs. Practicing self-compassion and patience is also important during these times, as it recognizes that healing is a continuous process with ups and downs.

In summary, the cookbook facilitates the eczema healing journey by documenting progress, setting baseline measurements, keeping a food and symptom log, recognizing non-scale triumphs, celebrating milestones, and staying inspired through plateaus and setbacks. Individuals who prioritize these themes can improve their dietary interventions for eczema control while also cultivating a sense of empowerment and resilience in navigating their health and well-being.

Healing from eczema demands more than just temporary solutions; long-term health and well-being necessitate a holistic approach. Adopting a diet that promotes your body's natural healing processes is an important part of maintaining your eczema treatment journey. This includes identifying trigger foods that aggravate your eczema symptoms and introducing anti-inflammatory and nutrient-dense foods into your diet.

In the Eczema Healing Diet Cookbook, you'll find tasty and nutritious foods that not only relieve symptoms but also promote overall health and vitality. These meals are intended to be consumed as part of a well-balanced diet that nourishes the body from the inside.

Furthermore, continuing your eczema recovery path necessitates persistence and dedication. Even if your symptoms begin to improve, you must adhere to your recovery plan. This includes adhering to the cookbook's food instructions while also embracing other healthy behaviors such as regular exercise, stress management strategies, and appropriate sleep.

In addition, being connected to a supportive group can be quite beneficial in your eczema healing path. A support network can help you stay motivated and accountable, whether through online forums, support groups, or discussing your experiences with friends and family.

Finally, sustaining your eczema healing path entails long-term lifestyle adjustments that benefit your entire health and well-being. You may maintain your progress and thrive by following a nourishing diet, sticking to your healing procedure, and connecting with others who understand your path.

Incorporating anti-inflammatory items into your diet is also a crucial long-term success approach. These nutrients reduce inflammation in the body, which can help relieve eczema symptoms and prevent flare-ups. The cookbook has recipes that are high in anti-inflammatory elements like fruits, vegetables, whole grains, and healthy fats, making it simple to incorporate these items into your everyday diet.

Furthermore, regular skincare habits are critical for keeping healthy skin and avoiding eczema flare-ups. This includes using gentle, fragrance-free skin care products, hydrating on a regular basis, and staying away from harsh chemicals or irritants that can aggravate symptoms.

The cookbook may also include ideas and recipes for homemade skincare cures that use natural substances to calm and nourish the skin.

Finally, implementing stress management practices and prioritizing self-care are critical for long-term eczema control. Stress can cause eczema flare-ups, so learning how to relax and unwind will help keep symptoms at bay. The cookbook may recommend ways to include stress-relieving activities into your daily routine, such as meditation, yoga, or spending time in nature.

Implementing these long-term success and maintenance tactics will allow you to effectively control your eczema symptoms and enjoy healthy, beautiful skin for many years to come.

CHAPTER TWELVE

Eczema recovery is not a one-size-fits-all process; your healing plan must be evaluated and adjusted on a continuous basis to match your changing needs.

The Eczema Healing Diet Cookbook provides instructions on how to examine and change your healing plan as needed to ensure sustained development and success.

Staying tuned in to your body's signals and responses to various foods and lifestyle circumstances is a key part of renewing your recovery program.

Your eczema triggers may fluctuate as your body changes and matures, necessitating an adjustment to your food and skincare routine. The cookbook may include tools like meal diaries or symptom trackers to help you track your progress and discover any changes or patterns that need to be adjusted.

Furthermore, engaging with healthcare professionals such as dermatologists, dietitians, or allergists can provide significant insights and advice on how to improve your healing routine. These professionals can assist you in identifying any underlying health issues or nutritional deficiencies that may be causing your eczema symptoms and recommending appropriate treatments.

Furthermore, testing with various dietary methods or lifestyle changes will help you figure out what works best for your specific circumstances. The cookbook may recommend alternative therapies like acupuncture, herbal remedies, or stress management practices to supplement your healing journey and promote general well-being.

Finally, evaluating and changing your healing routine as needed is critical to ensuring long-term success in eczema treatment. By remaining proactive and receptive to your body's changing demands, you may maintain your health and enjoy clear, healthy skin for many years.

Cultivating a Healthy and Resilient Mindset

Healing from eczema needs more than simply addressing physical symptoms; it also necessitates building a health and resilience mentality that promotes overall well-being. The Eczema Healing Diet Cookbook contains materials and information to help you establish a positive mindset that promotes healing and empowers you to overcome obstacles along the way.

Self-compassion and acceptance are important aspects of developing a healthy and resilient attitude. Living with eczema can be difficult, so it's vital to be kind to yourself and recognize your progress, no matter how tiny. The cookbook may include affirmations, journaling prompts, or mindfulness exercises to help you develop self-love and gratitude for your body's healing process.

Furthermore, viewing eczema as an opportunity for growth and self-discovery can help change your mindset from one of aggravation to one of empowerment. Instead of perceiving eczema as a setback, consider it a motivator for good change and personal improvement. The cookbook may contain encouraging anecdotes or testimonials from those who have successfully recovered from eczema, demonstrating that it is possible to overcome this condition and thrive.

Furthermore, growing resilience entails creating coping mechanisms for dealing with stress and adversity. This could include practicing relaxation techniques, setting limits, or getting help from loved ones. The cookbook may include materials for developing resilience and coping skills, allowing you to handle the ups and downs of your healing path with grace and power.

By building a healthy and resilient mindset, you can empower yourself to overcome hurdles, accept difficulties, and continue on your journey to recovery. With the appropriate attitude, you may turn your eczema experience into an opportunity for growth, healing, and self-discovery.

Sharing Knowledge and Experience with Others

Sharing your knowledge and experience with others who are going through similar struggles is one of the most effective methods to help your own healing path. The Eczema Healing Diet Cookbook provides encouragement and information on how to share your journey with others in a way that inspires and encourages them to take charge of their health and well-being.

Sharing your knowledge and experience with others can take various forms, ranging from participating in online forums and support groups to authoring blogs or articles on your eczema treatment. Sharing your story might provide hope, encouragement, and practical guidance to those who are dealing with eczema and looking for solutions.

Sharing your expertise and experience can also help raise awareness of eczema and encourage a better understanding and acceptance of the condition. By openly discussing your problems and achievements, you may help to reduce stigma and misconceptions about eczema and develop a more supportive and inclusive community for those afflicted by it.

Furthermore, sharing your journey with others can provide affirmation and connection, making you feel less isolated in your problems. Connecting with others who understand what you're going through can provide you with a sense of belonging and camaraderie, which can strengthen your determination and keep you motivated on your healing journey.

Finally, sharing your knowledge and experience with others is a wonderful method to pass it on and improve the lives of those around you. By sharing your story, you may inspire hope, encourage understanding, and create a supportive network for everyone affected by eczema.

Healing from eczema is a journey, not a destination, and it is critical to view it as a never-ending process of development, discovery, and transformation.

The Eczema Healing Diet Cookbook offers encouragement and support to help you approach your healing path with openness, resilience, and optimism.

Accepting the journey of eczema healing as a continual process entails accepting that healing requires time and patience. Although there may be ups and downs along the path, each setback is an opportunity for learning and progress. The cookbook may include resources such as guided meditations, affirmations, or inspiring quotes to help you remain cheerful and resilient in the face of adversity.

Furthermore, accepting the journey of eczema healing entails being willing to explore new tactics and strategies for managing your symptoms. What works for one person may not work for another, so be flexible and adaptable in your healing approach.

The cookbook may contain a range of recipes, suggestions, and procedures to help you tailor your healing routine to your specific needs and tastes.

Furthermore, embracing the journey of eczema healing entails growing compassion and appreciation for your body's tenacity and healing ability.

Instead of focusing on what's wrong with your skin, consider what's good with your body and enjoy your accomplishments thus far.

The cookbook may include techniques like gratitude writing or mindfulness exercises to help you create an appreciation and positive outlook.

By accepting the journey of eczema healing as an ongoing process, you may empower yourself to take control of your health and well-being and create a life that is vibrant, joyful, and full of possibilities. With the correct mindset and assistance, you can overcome the obstacles of eczema with grace and fortitude, emerging stronger, healthier, and more empowered than before.

Breakfast:

Blueberry oatmeal with almond milk

Ingredients: Rolled oats, almond milk, blueberries, and honey (optional).

Cook rolled oats in almond milk until smooth. If desired, sprinkle with honey and top with fresh blueberries.

Lunch:

Quinoa salad with roasted veggies.

Ingredients: Quinoa, mixed vegetables (bell peppers, zucchini, and carrots), olive oil, lemon juice, fresh herbs (parsley or basil), salt, and pepper.

Cook quinoa according to package directions. Roast mixed vegetables in olive oil, salt, and pepper until soft. Mix cooked quinoa with roasted veggies, fresh herbs, and a splash of lemon juice.

Dinner:

Baked salmon with steamed broccoli.

Ingredients: Salmon fillets, olive oil, lemon slices, garlic powder, salt, pepper, and broccoli.

Instructions: Preheat oven to 375°F (190°C). Put the salmon fillets on a baking pan lined with parchment paper. Drizzle with olive oil, then season with garlic powder, salt, and pepper. Finish with lemon slices. Bake for 12-15 minutes, or until the salmon is cooked through. Serve alongside steamed broccoli.

Snack:

Celery sticks with almond butter.

Ingredients: celery sticks and almond butter.

Spread almond butter on celery sticks for a crunchy and tasty snack.

Breakfast:

Avocado toast with cherry tomatoes.

Ingredients include whole grain bread, avocado, cherry tomatoes, olive oil, salt, pepper, and optional red pepper flakes.

Toast whole grain bread. Mash the avocado and distribute it atop the toast. Top with halved cherry tomatoes, olive oil, salt, pepper, and, if preferred, red pepper flakes.

Lunch:
Grilled chicken salad with mixed greens.

Ingredients: Chicken breast, mixed greens (e.g. spinach, arugula, kale), cucumber, bell pepper, cherry tomatoes, olive oil, balsamic vinegar, salt, and pepper.

Season chicken breast with salt and pepper and grill until cooked through. Grilled chicken is cut and served over a bed of mixed greens with sliced cucumber, bell pepper, and cherry tomatoes. Drizzle it with olive oil and balsamic vinegar.

Stir-fry vegetables with tofu.

Ingredients: Firm tofu, mixed vegetables (e.g. broccoli, bell peppers, snap peas), olive oil, soy sauce, garlic, ginger, sesame oil, and cooked brown rice.

To prepare the tofu, press it to remove excess moisture before cutting it into cubes. In a skillet, heat olive oil and stir in the minced garlic and ginger. Cook tofu cubes until golden brown. Add the mixed vegetables and cook until tender. Season with sesame oil and soy sauce. Serve over cooked brown rice.

Smoothie with mixed berries.

Ingredients include mixed berries (e.g. strawberries, blueberries, raspberries), almond milk, plain Greek yogurt, and optional

Instructions: Combine berries, almond milk, and plain Greek yogurt until smooth. If desired, sweeten with honey.

Chia Seed Pudding with Mango

Ingredients: Chia seeds, almond milk, mango, honey (optional).

For a thicker consistency, combine chia seeds and almond milk and refrigerate overnight. If desired, serve with diced mango and a drizzle of honey.

Brown Rice Sushi Rolls with Avocado and Cucumber.

Ingredients: Sushi rice, nori sheets, avocado, cucumber, rice vinegar, soy sauce (reduced sodium), wasabi (optional), and pickled ginger.

Cook sushi rice according to package directions and season with rice vinegar. Place a nori sheet on a bamboo sushi mat. Spread a thin layer of sushi rice across the nori sheet, leaving a border at the top. Add the sliced avocado and cucumber. Make a tight roll with the sushi mat. Cut into pieces and serve with wasabi, soy sauce, and pickled ginger.

Now, let us outline a 30-day meal plan:

Week 1:

Day 1:

Oatmeal with blueberries and almond milk.

Quinoa salad with roasted vegetables.

Baked salmon with steamed broccoli.

Celery sticks with almond butter.

Day 2:

Avocado Toast with Cherry Tomatoes.

Grilled Chicken Salad with Mixed Greens

Recipe: Vegetable Stir-Fry with Tofu.

Mixed Berries Smoothie (S)

Continue this pattern for the remainder of Week 1, alternating between the offered breakfast, lunch, dinner, and snack choices.

Week 2-4:

You can follow the Week 1 meal plan or mix and match the dishes above to provide variety while maintaining a balanced diet ideal for someone with dermatitis. Remember to consume enough of fruits, vegetables, whole grains, lean proteins, and healthy fats in your daily meals. Encourage drinking plenty of water and avoiding foods that can worsen eczema symptoms.

Adjust the portion proportions and ingredients to suit your specific preferences and dietary requirements. Also, always speak with a healthcare practitioner or trained nutritionist before making large dietary changes, especially if you have a specific health issue, such as eczema.

Conclusion:

In the Eczema Healing Diet Cookbook, we set out on a quest to regain control of our health and well-being in the face of eczema. This cookbook provides a guiding light for people navigating the complexity of eczema management by delving deeply into sustenance, perseverance, and self-discovery.

We have armed ourselves with the tools needed to embark on a transformative route toward recovery by exploring the principles of sustaining our healing journey, applying long-term success methods, and creating a mentality of health and resilience. From identifying trigger foods to accepting eczema healing as a never-ending process, each thought contributes to our quest for gorgeous skin and healthy health.

Furthermore, by sharing our knowledge and experiences with others, we not only empower ourselves but also help to build a community of support and understanding. Open discourse and compassionate outreach help to break down boundaries and develop a feeling of community that enriches us all.

As we come to the end of our examination of the Eczema Healing Diet Cookbook, let us embrace the knowledge gained from these pages and embark on our healing journey with newfound vigor and purpose. May this cookbook be a beacon of hope and inspiration, guiding us to a future full of health, happiness, and limitless possibilities.

THE END